LASER SKIN RESURFACING FOR BEGINNERS

Comprehensive Guide To Techniques, Benefits, And Essential Tips For Safe And Effective Rejuvenation

DR SAWYER DIEGO

DISCLAMER

Nothing in this book should be interpreted as medical advice; it is meant exclusively for educational reasons. Regarding their specific health issues and treatment options, readers are urged to speak with licensed healthcare professionals. The publisher and author disclaim all liability for any errors or omissions in the material provided, as well as for any negative effects that may arise from using or abusing the information. Although every attempt has been taken to guarantee that the material in this book is correct as of the date of publishing, new research may have superseded some of the content because medical knowledge is always changing. It is recommended that readers confirm the most recent medical recommendations and guidelines. The reader of this book undertakes to release the author and publisher from any claims or liabilities resulting from the use of this information, and understands and accepts the inherent risks connected with healthcare decisions.

TABLE OF CONTENTS

ABOUT THE BOOK

"Laser Skin Resurfacing for Beginners" delves into the complexities of laser skin resurfacing, providing a thorough exploration from its fundamental principles to practical applications and future trends. It is an invaluable resource for anyone considering or curious about enhancing their skin through advanced cosmetic procedures.

This guide provides readers with an insightful introduction to the concept of laser skin resurfacing, explaining its advantages and identifying its target audience. Whether your goal is to treat specific dermatological concerns, reduce scars, or rejuvenate aging skin, it gives you the knowledge you need to make wise decisions.

The book walks readers through important phases of the laser resurfacing process, beginning with a thorough explanation of the procedure itself. It goes over the mechanics of how lasers interact with skin tissues, explains the differences between ablative and non-ablative treatments, and outlines the typical outcomes. Throughout, safety is emphasized, and readers are given instructions on pre-treatment preparations, such as skin evaluations, consultations with cosmetic surgeons or dermatologists, and skincare regimens that are required.

The book offers a comforting synopsis of what to expect on procedure day, anesthetic considerations, and a detailed explanation of the treatment process. Post-treatment care instructions are meticulously detailed, guaranteeing maximum healing and long-term skin health.

Every detail, from managing immediate aftercare to shielding skin from sun exposure and identifying potential risks, is addressed with care to assist the reader through their healing process.

Foreseeing readers' worries, the book includes a section devoted to discussing typical side effects and how to effectively manage them. It also covers long-term consequences and when to seek medical attention for unexpected reactions, giving readers the knowledge they need to confidently navigate their recovery.

When it comes to the financial side, the guide looks at how much treatment costs, what affects pricing, what financing options are available, and whether insurance coverage is necessary? It also helps with choosing a qualified provider by providing advice on how to look up clinics, assess credentials, and use patient reviews as a guide.

Since not everyone is a good candidate for laser resurfacing, the book also looks at other options, weighing the benefits and drawbacks of each to help readers make decisions that are in line with their skincare objectives.

 Finally, it looks ahead at potential laser technology trends and future developments, highlighting the changing field of cosmetic dermatology and advising readers to keep up to date on new developments.

"Laser Skin Resurfacing for Beginners" equips readers with the knowledge, confidence, and awareness of their skincare needs to approach cosmetic procedures with clarity and confidence. It is more than just a guide; it is a companion on the path to healthier, rejuvenated skin.

CHAPTER ONE

LASER SKIN RESURFACING OVERVIEW

WHAT ARE SKIN RESURFACING USING LASERS?

A cosmetic procedure called laser skin resurfacing aims to rejuvenate the skin by treating different types of skin imperfections. By precisely removing damaged skin cells layer by layer and stimulating the growth of new, healthy skin cells, this treatment uses focused laser energy to target specific layers of the skin to improve texture, reduce wrinkles, and diminish scars or irregularities in pigmentation. The result is skin that is smoother, firmer and looks younger.

A numbing cream may be applied to minimize discomfort during the procedure, which consists of applying the laser device over the targeted areas and having a dermatologist or trained specialist assess your skin type and concerns to determine the most appropriate laser treatment. The laser produces controlled pulses of light that penetrate the skin, either ablating (removing) the outer layers or heating the underlying skin tissues to promote regeneration. Recovery time varies depending on the intensity of the treatment, ranging from a few days of redness and peeling to several weeks for more aggressive treatments.

The texture and appearance of the patient's skin usually improve gradually over the weeks that follow the procedure; multiple sessions may be necessary for best results, particularly for deeper skin concerns like deep wrinkles or acne scars; laser skin resurfacing is a flexible treatment that can be used on a variety of skin types and concerns; it offers customizable options that meet specific needs and desired results.

ADVANTAGES OF SKIN RESURFACING WITH LASER

To achieve a more youthful complexion without resorting to invasive surgery, laser skin resurfacing is a popular option due to its many benefits, one of which is its effectiveness in reducing signs of aging, such as fine lines, wrinkles, and age spots. Additionally, because laser treatments stimulate collagen production and promote skin regeneration, the result is smoother, firmer skin with improved elasticity.

Furthermore, by focusing on the damaged skin layers and encouraging the formation of new, healthy tissue, laser resurfacing can effectively treat scars resulting from acne or injuries.

This can greatly improve skin texture and minimize the visibility of scars, improving overall skin tone and clarity. Lastly, the precision of the treatment allows dermatologists to target specific areas of concern without affecting the surrounding skin, minimizing the risk of adverse effects.

In addition, laser skin resurfacing procedures are generally quick and easy, with little downtime after the procedure.

Depending on how strong the procedure is, patients may have temporary redness, swelling, or peeling, but these effects usually go away in a few days to a week. Newer laser treatments are gentler while still being effective, providing patients with better comfort and quicker recovery periods.

WHO IS THIS BOOK SUITABLE FOR?

This book about laser skin resurfacing is meant for people who want to learn about cosmetic procedures that are intended to improve the appearance of skin and address common issues like wrinkles, scars, and uneven pigmentation. It is especially helpful for people who are thinking about laser treatments but aren't sure if they're a good fit for them or what the process entails. Adults of all ages who want to improve the texture of their skin, lessen signs of aging, or look better overall can benefit from reading this book.

This book offers thorough insights into the advantages, factors to consider, and anticipated results of laser resurfacing. It is intended for people who want to make well-informed decisions about their skincare routine and investigate non-surgical options to achieve smoother, more youthful-looking skin.

By outlining the procedures, anticipated recovery times, and possible outcomes, it hopes to arm readers with the knowledge they need to confidently navigate their skincare journey.

HOW TO UTILIZE THIS MANUAL

Readers are advised to begin by familiarizing themselves with the basics of laser treatments; including how they operate and what skin concerns they address, to get the most out of this guide on laser skin resurfacing.

Next, learn about the various types of laser resurfacing techniques that are available, ranging from ablative to non-ablative options, and the advantages of each.

After being familiar with the available treatment options, readers can dive into the details of getting ready for a laser procedure, such as skincare routines before the procedure, advice for consultations, and what to anticipate during the procedure; comprehensive post-procedure care is also included, guiding readers through the healing process and providing advice to maximize outcomes and minimize discomfort.

By following the recommendations outlined in each section, readers can approach laser skin resurfacing with confidence, knowing they have the knowledge and tools to make informed decisions and effectively achieve their skincare goals. Practical insights and expert advice are used throughout the guide to help readers navigate every step of their journey toward healthier, rejuvenated skin.

TAKING SAFETY FACTORS INTO ACCOUNT

To ensure a positive treatment experience and optimal results, there are several safety factors to take into account before undergoing laser skin resurfacing. The first is that you should choose a qualified and experienced cosmetic surgeon or dermatologist; make sure to check their credentials and ask about their experience with laser treatments, particularly the kind of laser technology they use and whether it is appropriate for your concerns and skin type.

It's important to disclose any allergies, skin sensitivities, or previous skin treatments to your provider to prevent potential complications during or after the procedure.

You should also discuss with your healthcare provider any current medical conditions or medications. Certain health conditions or medications may affect your eligibility for laser treatments or require adjustments to the procedure.

To achieve satisfactory results from laser skin resurfacing, it is important to understand the expected outcomes and realistic expectations before beginning the procedure.

Additionally, to maximize the effectiveness and safety of the procedure, adhere to pre-treatment guidelines provided by your provider, such as avoiding sun exposure, stopping certain skincare products, or preparing the skin as instructed. These steps should be taken before beginning laser skin resurfacing.

CHAPTER TWO

COMPREHENDING SKIN RESURFACING

INTRODUCTION

Using laser technology to remove damaged skin layers, laser skin resurfacing is a cosmetic procedure that improves the texture and appearance of the skin. It is a common way to reduce wrinkles, scars, blemishes, and other irregularities on the skin, leaving the skin smoother and more youthful-looking. It can be customized to target specific concerns, making it a flexible option in dermatology and aesthetic medicine.

By precisely removing layers of skin tissue with a laser beam, laser skin resurfacing stimulates the skin's natural healing response and stimulates the production of new collagen and elastin fibers, which are essential proteins that give the skin structure and elasticity and help to give the appearance of younger skin.

The laser treatment's depth and intensity can be adjusted to achieve different results depending on the condition being treated and the desired outcome, so each patient receives a customized treatment plan.

Individuals who are thinking about getting laser skin resurfacing should speak with a licensed dermatologist or cosmetic surgeon to evaluate their skin type and choose the best course of action. Having a basic understanding of the principles underlying laser skin resurfacing and its possible advantages empowers people to make well-informed choices regarding improving the appearance and health of their skin.

WHAT IS THE PROCESS OF LASER SKIN RESURFACING?

By vaporizing the targeted skin cells, concentrated light beams are used in laser skin resurfacing to remove skin layers precisely, layer by layer. This process minimizes downtime and lowers the risk of complications by allowing for the controlled removal of damaged skin while leaving the surrounding tissue intact. The laser emits short pulses of high-energy light that are absorbed by the water and chromophores (pigments) in the skin.

Ablative lasers, like carbon dioxide (CO2) or erbium lasers, remove thin layers of skin to reveal healthier, smoother skin beneath; non-ablative lasers, like fractional lasers, target deeper layers of skin without removing the outer layer, stimulating collagen production and improving skin tone and texture over time. These two types of lasers are commonly used in skin resurfacing procedures.

Recovery times vary depending on the type of laser used and the extent of treatment; some patients experience redness, swelling, and mild discomfort for a few days to a week following the procedure. The procedure is usually performed under local anesthesia or sedation in a medical office or dermatology clinic.

KINDS OF LASER THERAPY

Treatments for sun damage, deep wrinkles, and scars can all be effectively treated with laser skin resurfacing. Ablative lasers, like fractional CO2 lasers, work by vaporizing damaged skin cells and promoting the production of collagen. Although they have dramatic effects, they may take longer to heal than non-ablative options.

Non-ablative laser treatments, such as fractional lasers and pulsed dye lasers, are less invasive and require less downtime, making them ideal for patients seeking gradual improvement in skin tone and mild to moderate signs of aging. These treatments work by targeting underlying skin layers to promote collagen growth and improve skin texture.

Fractional lasers, in particular, allow for targeted treatment of specific areas with minimal risk of side effects and guarantee natural-looking results by creating microscopic treatment zones within the skin while leaving surrounding tissue untouched to speed up healing and reduce recovery time.

The most effective and safest laser treatment plan customized to each patient's needs will be determined by taking into account aspects including skin type, intended objectives, and the severity of skin issues. Consulting with a knowledgeable dermatologist or cosmetic surgeon is vital.

THE DISTINCTIONS BETWEEN NON-ABLATIVE AND ABLATIVE LASERS

Choosing between ablative and non-ablative lasers is a crucial distinction in laser skin resurfacing, as each has its advantages and disadvantages. Ablative lasers, like CO_2 or erbium lasers, work by vaporizing superficial layers of skin to stimulate collagen production and improve skin texture. Although they can treat deep wrinkles, scars, and irregular pigmentation, they may require longer recovery times than non-ablative options.

Non-ablative lasers, like fractional lasers and pulsed dye lasers, are less invasive and require less downtime, making them ideal for patients seeking mild signs of aging and subtle improvements in skin texture. These lasers target deeper layers of skin without damaging the outer layer, promoting collagen growth and enhancing skin tone.

Ablative lasers offer more dramatic results with a single procedure, but careful post-procedure care is necessary to manage healing and minimize risks. Non-ablative lasers provide gradual improvement with multiple sessions and are suitable for patients looking to enhance skin texture without lengthy recovery periods. The choice between ablative and non-ablative lasers depends on factors such as the severity of skin concerns, desired downtime, and patient expectations.

People can make well-informed decisions about laser skin resurfacing by being aware of the differences between ablative and non-ablative lasers, which help to ensure optimal results according to their skin type and aesthetic goals.

AN OVERVIEW OF THE ANTICIPATED OUTCOMES

Ablative lasers usually offer immediate improvements in skin texture and tone by removing damaged outer layers and stimulating collagen production. Patients may experience smoother skin, reduced wrinkles, and diminished scars following treatment, with continued improvement over several months as new collagen forms. The results of laser skin resurfacing vary depending on the type of laser used, the depth of treatment, and individual skin characteristics.

Through a series of treatments, patients may notice subtle improvements in skin texture, reduced pore size, and enhanced overall skin appearance. Non-ablative lasers, like fractional lasers, are effective for maintaining youthful skin and addressing early signs of aging with minimal downtime. By targeting deeper skin layers and promoting collagen growth without disrupting the surface, these lasers deliver gradual enhancement.

While individual results may vary depending on skin condition, treatment intensity, and post-procedure care, patients need to manage their expectations. Patients should adhere to the skincare and sun protection recommendations made by their cosmetic surgeon or dermatologist to maximize and prolong the benefits of laser treatment.

Patients can express their problems, expectations, and goals for laser skin resurfacing by consulting with a skilled skincare practitioner. This ensures a customized treatment plan that safely and efficiently accomplishes desired aesthetic effects.

CHAPTER THREE
GETTING READY FOR THERAPY
CONSULTATION WITH A COSMETIC SURGEON OR DERMATOLOGIST

It's important to arrange a consultation with a dermatologist or cosmetic surgeon who specializes in skin treatments before beginning laser skin resurfacing. In this initial appointment, the specialist will examine your desired areas of treatment (fine lines, wrinkles, acne scars, sun damage), as well as your medical history and concerns regarding the procedure. They will also determine the best laser treatment approach based on these evaluations.

In addition to explaining the various types of laser resurfacing options available, such as ablative or non-ablative lasers, and recommending the most effective treatment based on your skin type and condition, the dermatologist or surgeon will also provide detailed instructions on how to prepare for the procedure, including any necessary skincare routines or medications to avoid before treatment, during the consultation. You should use this time to ask any questions you may have about the procedure.

Following your consultation, you ought to have a comprehensive understanding of the possible outcomes and recovery times associated with laser skin resurfacing. This individualized approach guarantees that the treatment plan is customized to your requirements, increasing the likelihood of attaining desired results while lowering risks.

ASSESSING THE TYPE AND CONDITION OF SKIN

Your dermatologist or cosmetic surgeon will carefully assess your skin's texture, tone, elasticity, and any existing concerns, such as acne, pigmentation issues, or fine lines. This evaluation helps determine the appropriate laser wavelength, intensity, and treatment approach best suited to address your specific skin issues. To effectively achieve the desired cosmetic improvements, consideration will be given to factors such as skin sensitivity, tendency to develop scars, and recent sun exposure. Based on this information, the type of laser to use—ablative, which removes outer layers of skin, or non-ablative, which stimulates collagen production without damaging the surface—will be chosen.

Your dermatologist will also go over reasonable expectations based on the state of your skin now and the desired results of the procedure. This thorough assessment guarantees that the laser skin resurfacing procedure is safe and customized to your specific skin needs, maximizing the chance of having smoother, younger-looking skin.

PRE-MEDICATION SKIN CARE PROTOCOLS

Your dermatologist will provide you with detailed instructions on a pre-treatment skin care regimen designed to maximize results and minimize potential side effects. Generally, this regimen entails gentle cleansing with a mild, non-irritating cleanser to remove impurities and excess oil without stripping the skin's natural moisture barrier. Proper skin preparation is essential for ensuring both an effective treatment and a smooth recovery following laser skin resurfacing.

Apart from cleaning, your dermatologist might advise against using specific skincare products and medications that might aggravate your skin or cause problems with the laser treatment.

It's critical to adhere to these recommendations to lower the possibility of negative reactions and guarantee that the laser can effectively target your skin imperfections.

In addition, by following the suggested pre-treatment skincare routine, you can maximize the benefits of laser skin resurfacing and attain smoother, more radiant skin with the least amount of discomfort. Make sure you stay properly hydrated by drinking lots of water and using a moisturizer that is appropriate for your skin type.

SETTING OBJECTIVES AND CONTROLLING EXPECTATIONS

Setting clear and attainable goals with your dermatologist or cosmetic surgeon before laser skin resurfacing is crucial. The consultation process is a critical component in controlling expectations as it covers the procedure's limitations as well as possible outcomes based on your skin type, condition, and desired results.

Your healthcare provider will answer any questions you may have regarding recovery time, possible side effects, and the number of sessions needed to achieve optimal results, as well as the expected improvements in skin texture, tone, and overall appearance that can be achieved through laser resurfacing.

Establishing concrete objectives, like lessening the visibility of fine lines, increasing skin suppleness, or decreasing acne scars, helps to balance expectations and guarantees that you and your physician agree with the desired cosmetic results.

This cooperative approach promotes reasonable expectations and increases satisfaction with the outcomes of laser skin resurfacing.

RECOGNIZING POSSIBLE DANGERS AND SIDE EFFECTS

Although laser skin resurfacing is usually safe and effective, it is important to be aware of the possible risks and side effects that come with the procedure; your cosmetic surgeon or dermatologist will go over these in the consultation to minimize any unexpected consequences and ensure that you give informed consent.

Depending on the extent of the treatment, common side effects of laser resurfacing include temporary redness, swelling, and mild discomfort akin to a sunburn, which usually goes away in a few days to weeks. Less common but potentially serious side effects include infection, scarring, or changes in skin pigmentation, especially if post-treatment care instructions are not carefully followed.

Your healthcare provider will discuss post-treatment care instructions, such as when to resume normal activities and avoid sun exposure to prevent complications and maximize results, to minimize risks. These instructions will include the use of gentle cleansers, moisturizers, and sunscreen to protect your skin during the healing process.

Knowing the possible dangers and adverse effects of laser skin resurfacing can help you make well-informed decisions about your skin care regimen and be assured that you will achieve smoother, more youthful-looking skin with the least amount of risk.

CHAPTER FOUR
THE DAY OF PROCEDURE
WHAT TO ANTICIPATE FROM THE PROCESS

A dermatologist or cosmetic surgeon will typically evaluate your skin condition and discuss your goals during your consultation. On the day of the procedure, you will arrive at the clinic and be made comfortable in the treatment room, where the area to be treated will be thoroughly cleaned and your eyes will be protected with safety shields. Laser skin resurfacing is a precise cosmetic procedure intended to rejuvenate the skin by reducing wrinkles, scars, and other irregularities.

After all is in place, the laser will be adjusted based on your skin type and the particular concerns that need to be addressed. You might experience a warming sensation as the laser targets the problematic areas of your skin. The length of the procedure will depend on the size of the treatment area and the complexity of the issues that need to be addressed.

Following the treatment, the skin may be soothed with a cooling ointment or soothing mask.

GETTING READY: MENTAL AND PHYSICAL

To guarantee a smooth and successful procedure, you should be mentally and physically prepared for laser skin resurfacing. You should discuss any worries you may have with your healthcare provider before the procedure and try to be realistic about the results and potential downtime. You should also physically prepare by adhering to any pre-procedure instructions that your healthcare provider provides, such as avoiding certain medications, skincare products, or activities that could affect the skin's sensitivity or healing process.

You will maximize the benefits and reduce the risks associated with laser skin resurfacing by mentally preparing and following physical guidelines. On the day of the procedure, make sure your skin is clean and free of any makeup or lotions. Dress comfortably and make arrangements for someone to accompany you if necessary, especially if sedation is involved. Prepare your home environment for post-treatment recovery by stocking up on recommended skin care products and making sure a calm, restful space to recuperate.

COMFORT-ORIENTED ANESTHESIA OPTIONS

For lighter treatments, topical anesthesia in the form of numbing creams or gels may be applied to the skin before the procedure. This helps dull any discomfort during the laser application. During laser skin resurfacing, a variety of anesthesia options are available to ensure your comfort throughout the procedure. The choice of anesthesia depends on the depth of treatment and your pain tolerance.

In certain cases, particularly for extensive treatments or those involving deeper skin layers, sedation or general anesthesia may be recommended. This option allows you to remain unconscious or deeply relaxed during the procedure, making it more manageable and pain-free. Your healthcare provider will discuss the most suitable anesthesia option based on your individual needs and the planned extent of treatment. For more intense treatments, local anesthesia may be injected into the treatment area to completely numb the skin. This ensures you remain comfortable and relaxed throughout the procedure.

COMPREHENSIVE PROCESS OVERVIEW

Laser skin resurfacing is a step-by-step process that involves several important steps to achieve the best results while maintaining patient safety. Firstly, the treatment area needs to be thoroughly cleaned to remove any debris, oils, or makeup that could interfere with the laser's effectiveness. Secondly, numbing cream, local anesthetic, or sedation, depending on the type of anesthesia selected, will be applied to ensure your comfort throughout the procedure.

Following the onset of anesthesia, the laser device is calibrated to the proper settings for your skin type and the particular issues being addressed. The laser is then directed over the skin, producing precise light pulses that target and remove damaged skin cells layer by layer, promoting the production of collagen and revealing healthier, smoother skin beneath. The length of the procedure depends on the size of the treatment area and the complexity of the issues being addressed.

A cooling mask or soothing ointment may be applied to the treated skin after the laser passes are finished to minimize discomfort and encourage healing. Your healthcare provider will give you detailed instructions on what to do at home after the procedure, including how to take medication, take care of your skin, and what side effects to be aware of while you recover.

INSTRUCTIONS FOR POST-TREATMENT CARE

Following the recommended post-treatment care instructions is essential for optimizing results and reducing complications following laser skin resurfacing. Your healthcare provider will give you specific instructions based on your needs and the degree of resurfacing; in general, you will be told to keep the treated area clean and moisturized using gentle skincare products.

Attend follow-up appointments as scheduled to monitor the healing progress of your skin and address any concerns promptly. Depending on the depth of the treatment, you may experience redness, swelling, or mild discomfort, which can be managed with prescribed medications or over-the-counter pain relievers. Avoid sun exposure and wear broad-spectrum sunscreen with SPF 30 or higher to protect the newly treated skin from UV damage.

After laser skin resurfacing, you should be patient during the healing period because the skin heals and regenerates over several weeks.

CHAPTER FIVE

FOLLOWING TREATMENT CARE

QUICK AFTERCARE INSTRUCTIONS

Following the instructions for immediate aftercare following laser skin resurfacing is critical for the best healing and outcomes. First and foremost, you should keep the treated area clean and dry to avoid infection. Your dermatologist may advise using a light moisturizer or ointment to help the skin heal and stay hydrated. Finally, you should refrain from touching or picking at the treated area to prevent irritation and possible scarring.

In addition, following your doctor's instructions regarding the use of cold compresses or pain relievers can help to minimize swelling and discomfort during the healing process. It's common for the skin to feel tight or itchy during the healing process; however, refrain from scratching to avoid further complications.

To attain the intended results of laser skin resurfacing, protect the skin throughout the early healing phase. Finally, adhere to any special advice given by your dermatologist regarding skincare products and cosmetics use.

HANDLING PAIN AND REDNESS

Your dermatologist may advise using prescribed pain relievers or anti-inflammatory medications to effectively manage any discomfort. After laser skin resurfacing, you may experience mild to moderate discomfort at first, which can be relieved by applying cool compresses or ice packs to the treated area.

Gentle skincare is key to reducing redness and inflammation. Stay hydrated to support the healing process and minimize redness over time. Use a mild cleanser and follow with a soothing moisturizer recommended by your dermatologist. Steer clear of harsh cleansers or exfoliants that could irritate the sensitive skin.

Sun protection helps to maintain the results of laser skin resurfacing and prevents pigmentation issues. It is important to protect the treated skin from UV rays as they can exacerbate redness and delay healing. Consider wearing a broad-spectrum sunscreen with SPF 30 or higher daily, even on cloudy days, and reapply as directed.

KEEPING TREATED SKIN SAFE FROM THE SUN

After laser skin resurfacing, it is critical to protect your skin from the sun to avoid complications and achieve the best possible results. Direct sunlight can cause hyperpigmentation, prolonged redness, and even scarring on the treated areas of your skin. To protect your skin, generously apply a broad-spectrum sunscreen with SPF 30 or higher, and reapply it every two hours, especially if you are outdoors.

To further protect yourself from UV rays, wear protective clothing like long sleeves, wide-brimmed hats, and sunglasses.

Avoid being outside between the hours of 10 a.m. and 4 p.m., when the sun is at its strongest. If you must be outside, find shade whenever you can, and reapply sunscreen frequently.

Continue to prioritize sun protection even after the initial phase of recovery to preserve the outcomes of your laser skin resurfacing treatment and to keep your skin healthy. Adherent sun protection techniques are crucial during the healing period and beyond.

TRACKING THE HEALING PROCESS

Following laser skin resurfacing, it is helpful to watch the healing process to spot any potential problems early on. You may experience some initial soreness, swelling, and redness, but these are normal healing side effects that should gradually go away as the days go by.

During this period, proper wound care and hygiene are crucial to minimize the risk of complications.

Keep an eye out for any signs of infection, such as increased redness, warmth, or pus-like discharge. Contact your dermatologist as soon as possible for further evaluation and guidance if you notice these symptoms or if the pain worsens instead of getting better.

By actively tracking your skin's healing progress, you can guarantee a smooth recovery and get the best results from laser skin resurfacing. Pay attention to how your skin reacts to treatments and products that your dermatologist recommends. Modify your skin care regimen as necessary to support healing and maintain skin health.

WHEN TO MAKE FOLLOW-UP CONSULTATIONS

Following laser skin resurfacing, it is important to know when to schedule follow-up appointments to monitor healing and address any concerns. Your dermatologist will usually advise when to schedule your first follow-up visit, which should happen within the first week following the procedure. During this visit, they will evaluate your healing progress, answer any questions you may have, and recommend additional treatments if needed.

Your dermatologist may recommend additional laser sessions or complementary treatments to improve the results of your initial procedure. Follow-up appointments can also be used to discuss any changes in your skin's condition or concerns regarding the healing process. Following your procedure, you may be scheduled for follow-up appointments to monitor long-term results and make any necessary adjustments to your skincare regimen.

At follow-up appointments, you can make sure you receive comprehensive care and the best possible outcome from your laser skin resurfacing procedure. Your dermatologist can monitor your progress, assess the efficacy of the treatment, and provide you with customized recommendations for ongoing skin care.

CHAPTER SIX
POSSIBLE DANGERS AND ISSUES
TYPICAL SIDE EFFECTS FOLLOWING THERAPY

Several side effects are common following laser skin resurfacing as your skin heals and adjusts to the treatment. Redness and swelling are the most common side effects, and they usually go away in a few days to a week. Your skin may also feel warm or sensitive, similar to a mild sunburn. During this time, it's important to keep your treated skin moisturized and out of direct sunlight to speed up the healing process.

While mild itching or discomfort may occur during the healing process, some patients may notice temporary changes in their skin's pigmentation, either lighter or darker patches, which usually go away as new skin cells regenerate. It is important to adhere to the post-treatment care instructions that your dermatologist or healthcare provider provides to minimize these effects and promote optimal healing. Most of the time, these side effects are manageable and resolve without complications, resulting in smoother, more youthful-looking skin in the long run.

SIGNS OF DIFFICULTIES TO BE AWARE OF

While laser skin resurfacing is generally safe, some warning signs should raise red flags and necessitate medical attention. These include severe pain that lasts longer than anticipated, excessive swelling or redness that gets worse instead of better, and the formation of pus or unusual discharge from treated areas. These symptoms could indicate infection, which requires immediate evaluation and treatment by a medical professional.

Any new or worsening skin discoloration, especially if it extends beyond the treated area, should also be evaluated by a dermatologist. Additionally, if you experience fever or chills after treatment, you must seek medical advice promptly. These signs and prompt medical attention can help mitigate potential complications and ensure a successful recovery from laser skin resurfacing.

WAYS TO HANDLE UNEXPECTED RESPONSES

After laser skin resurfacing, there are a few important steps to take to manage any unexpected reactions that may arise. First, if you notice any increased redness or swelling, you should apply cool compresses gently to the treated area to help reduce these symptoms. Secondly, you should avoid picking or scratching at any scabs that may form because doing so can cause scarring and prolong healing.

Maintaining skin hydration and relieving irritation can also be achieved by keeping your skin well-hydrated with non-comedogenic products that your dermatologist has recommended. You should get in touch with your healthcare provider as soon as possible if you have severe or persistent symptoms, such as severe pain, significant swelling, or signs of infection.

They can offer advice on additional treatments or medications to help manage your symptoms and facilitate a speedy recovery. By taking these preventative steps and getting in touch with them as soon as you need to, you can maximize your results and feel confident when dealing with unanticipated reactions following laser skin resurfacing.

CONSEQUENCES OF LASER SKIN RESURFACING OVER TIME

Although laser skin resurfacing can result in significant improvements to the texture and appearance of the skin, it is important to understand the possible long-term effects to make an informed decision. Sun protection is especially important because treated skin often becomes more sensitive to sunlight over time. Erythematic, or persistent redness, can occur in some people, especially those with fair skin or sensitive skin. It usually goes away over time but may need to be maintained with ongoing skincare regimens designed for sensitive skin types.

Long-lasting improvements in skin tone and texture can also result in a more youthful and refreshed appearance overall.

Working closely with your dermatologist or healthcare provider ensures personalized care and ongoing monitoring of your skin's health and response to treatment. By being aware of these potential long-term effects and putting appropriate skincare practices into practice, you can maximize the benefits of laser skin resurfacing and enjoy sustained improvements in skin quality and appearance. For those who are prone to skin conditions like acne or rosacea, laser skin resurfacing may provide extended relief from symptoms and reduce the frequency of flare-ups.

ASKING MEDICAL PROFESSIONALS FOR ASSISTANCE

Following laser skin resurfacing, if you have any worrisome symptoms or complications, you should get medical help right away for the best possible results. Dermatologists and other skincare specialists are qualified to assess and treat any problems that may develop during the healing phase and can provide customized guidance and treatment plans to effectively manage symptoms and avert complications.

In addition to prescribing medications to relieve discomfort, encourage healing, or prevent infection, your healthcare provider can evaluate the severity of symptoms, such as chronic pain, excessive swelling, or infection-related symptoms, and recommend appropriate interventions. They can also offer advice on sun protection techniques and post-treatment skincare routines to improve recovery and maintain long-term results.

To ensure that your skin responds positively to laser resurfacing and to address any emerging concerns promptly, schedule regular follow-up appointments with your healthcare provider.

CHAPTER SEVEN

FAQS REGARDING SKIN RESURFACING USING LASERS

IS SKIN RESURFACING WITH LASER SAFE FOR ALL?

All skin types and tones can benefit from laser skin resurfacing, but conditions like active acne, eczema, or infections may need to be treated before the procedure. Your medical history, current medications, and skin condition will be evaluated to ensure safety and effectiveness.

Most people can generally be considered candidates for laser skin resurfacing, but it's important to speak with a qualified dermatologist or cosmetic surgeon to determine your candidacy.

Overall, laser skin resurfacing is a safe option for improving skin texture, tone, and appearance when done under appropriate medical supervision. You may experience mild discomfort during the procedure, similar to a snapping sensation or warmth on the skin, but this can be managed with topical anesthesia or cooling techniques. Modern laser technologies have advanced significantly, minimizing risks such as pigmentation changes or scarring, especially when performed by experienced professionals. Sun protection and gentle skincare are crucial aftercare instructions to maximize healing and minimize potential side effects.

HOW MANY MEETINGS ARE USUALLY NEEDED?

The number of laser skin resurfacing sessions needed varies based on the type of laser used and the condition of your skin. One session may be enough to address mild to moderate concerns like wrinkles, fine lines, or uneven skin tone, while multiple sessions spaced several weeks apart may be necessary to address more severe conditions like deep wrinkles or acne scars.

Your doctor will evaluate your skin's condition and create a customized treatment plan during your initial consultation. The number of sessions that are recommended will depend on several factors, including the intensity of the laser, your skin's response to treatment, and your desired results. Each session lasts 30 minutes to an hour, during which time the laser energy is applied to specific areas of your skin to stimulate collagen production and rejuvenate the skin's surface.

It's important to carefully follow post-treatment care instructions to maximize results and minimize potential side effects.

Following the recommended treatment schedule and implementing a thorough skincare regimen can help you gradually achieve smoother, more youthful-looking skin. Following each session, you may experience redness, swelling, or mild discomfort, but these side effects usually go away after a few days.

WHAT MUST I AVERT FOLLOWING TREATMENT?

For optimal healing and results following laser skin resurfacing, there are a few things you must do. First, you should avoid direct sunlight and UV exposure for at least a week following the procedure; wear protective clothing and a hat when you're outside, and use a broad-spectrum sunscreen with an SPF of 30 or higher. Your skin may feel sensitive after the procedure, similar to mild sunburn.

For the first few days following treatment, stay out of hot baths, steam rooms, saunas, and intense exercise to minimize sweating and irritation. You should also avoid picking, scratching, or exfoliating the treated area because these actions can impede the healing process and raise the risk of complications like infection or hyperpigmentation. Instead, use the gentle cleansers and moisturizers that have been prescribed by your healthcare provider to soothe and hydrate the skin.

Additionally, until your skin has completely healed, stay away from harsh skincare products that contain glycolic acid, retinoids, or exfoliating agents. Instead, use gentle, non-irritating formulas that aid in the skin's healing and preserve its newly restored clarity and smoothness. By carefully adhering to these aftercare instructions, you can maximize the results of laser skin resurfacing and take pleasure in long-lasting enhancements in the texture and appearance of your skin.

CAN CERTAIN SKIN CONCERNS BE TREATED WITH LASER RESURFACING?

Whether you're bothered by fine lines, wrinkles, sun damage, acne scars, or uneven pigmentation, laser treatments can be customized to target and improve these areas. Different types of lasers, such as ablative and non-ablative, offer varying depths of penetration and treatment intensities to suit individual needs. Laser skin resurfacing is very versatile and can effectively address a wide range of specific skin concerns.

While non-ablative lasers like fractional lasers penetrate the skin in a fractionated pattern, sparing surrounding tissues while promoting healing and skin tightening, ablative lasers like CO2 or Erbium-YAG are best for treating deep wrinkles and scars by removing layers of damaged skin and stimulating collagen production in the dermis.

These treatments can also improve overall skin tone and texture, giving the appearance of more youthful and radiant skin.

Laser skin resurfacing is still a flexible and effective way to rejuvenate the skin, thanks to advancements in laser technology and customized treatment plans. However, before undergoing laser resurfacing, it is important to discuss your specific concerns and treatment goals with a qualified healthcare provider. They will evaluate your skin condition and recommend the most appropriate laser technology and treatment approach to achieve optimal results.

WHAT IS THE DURATION OF RESULTS?

In general, the effects of laser treatments can last anywhere from several months to several years, with proper maintenance and sun protection. The longevity of results from laser skin resurfacing varies depending on several factors, including the type of laser used, your skin's natural aging process, sun exposure, and skincare regimen.

Fine lines, wrinkles, and scars may appear diminished, and skin may feel smoother and more youthful immediately after treatment. You may notice an improvement in skin texture, tone, and overall clarity, which can continue to enhance over the following weeks as collagen production is stimulated and the skin heals.

If you want to extend the benefits of laser resurfacing, you should follow a regular skincare regimen that consists of gentle cleansers, moisturizers, and sunscreens. You can also prolong the rejuvenated appearance of your skin by avoiding excessive sun exposure and using sun protection measures like hats and daily sunscreen application.

Long-lasting improvements in skin texture and tone can be achieved by partnering with a skilled healthcare provider and adhering to their guidance for post-treatment care and maintenance. Although laser skin resurfacing produces noticeable results, individual outcomes may vary and periodic maintenance treatments may be recommended to sustain optimal skin health and appearance.

CHAPTER EIGHT

INSURANCE AND COST FACTORS

COMPREHENDING THE COST OF TREATMENT

The cost of laser skin resurfacing varies greatly depending on several factors. The extent of the treatment area is the most important factor, as larger areas or multiple treatment areas will naturally incur higher costs compared to smaller, more localized treatments. Other factors that affect the overall cost of laser skin resurfacing include the type of laser used and the specific technique used by the dermatologist or cosmetic surgeon. Finally, advanced laser technologies or specialized treatment methods may come at a premium price due to their efficacy and precision.

Geographical location can also affect treatment costs. Generally speaking, cosmetic procedures cost more in urban centers and higher-cost regions than in rural areas.

People thinking about laser skin resurfacing should look into local pricing trends and compare quotes from several providers. Knowing the breakdown of costs—which usually include consultation fees, procedure fees, anesthesia costs (if applicable), and post-procedure care expenses—allows them to make an informed decision.

Prospective patients can better prepare financially for their laser skin resurfacing journey by getting detailed cost estimates and talking about payment options up front.

When planning a budget for laser skin resurfacing, it's important to account for potential out-of-pocket costs, such as prescription drugs for pre-and post-procedure care and any necessary follow-up visits. Openness about costs and thorough financial planning guarantee that patients can start their treatment journey with assurance, knowing they have carefully considered all financial aspects.

VARIABLES IMPACTING THE COST

Prospective patients should be aware of the various factors that affect the cost of laser skin resurfacing procedures. The type of laser used for the procedure is one of the main determinants, as different lasers offer different levels of intensity and precision. Newer technologies often command higher costs due to their advanced capabilities and enhanced safety profiles. The specific condition being treated also plays a part in the pricing of laser skin resurfacing procedures; more severe cases of skin damage or aging may require more intensive treatment protocols, which may have an impact on overall pricing.

Furthermore, the location of the practice affects pricing dynamics. Practices located in metropolitan areas or upscale neighborhoods typically have higher overhead costs, which can translate into higher treatment prices. The experience and expertise of the dermatologist or cosmetic surgeon performing the procedure also have a significant impact on costs.

Practitioners with extensive training and a track record of successful outcomes may charge higher fees for their services.

Pricing varies depending on several patient-specific factors, including skin type, medical history, and desired treatment outcomes. Treatment plans that are customized to meet the specific needs of each patient may incur additional costs for follow-up appointments and personalized care. Those who are thinking about laser skin resurfacing should schedule a thorough consultation with a qualified provider to discuss these factors and receive a detailed cost estimate. Patients can make decisions that are in line with their financial capabilities and cosmetic goals by being aware of the subtleties of pricing determinants.

AVAILABLE FINANCING OPTIONS

The process of navigating the financial aspects of laser skin resurfacing can be made easier by looking into a variety of financing options that can accommodate a range of budgets and preferences.

 A lot of dermatology and cosmetic surgery practices offer flexible payment plans that can be tailored to the financial needs of their patients. These plans can allow for installment payments spread out over several months, which can help patients with the immediate financial burden of the procedure. Patients should ask questions about the terms, interest rates, and eligibility criteria of the financing options that are available during their initial consultation.

Examining these outside financing options can enable patients to receive treatment sooner rather than later without compromising their financial stability. In addition, healthcare financing companies and third-party lenders specialize in providing loans specifically for medical procedures like laser skin resurfacing. These lenders frequently offer competitive interest rates and repayment terms tailored to suit individual needs. Some practices may even partner with financing providers to streamline the application process and expedite approval for qualified applicants.

Additionally, some patients might choose to pay for laser skin resurfacing with healthcare savings accounts (HSAs) or flexible spending accounts (FSAs). These tax-advantaged accounts let people set aside pre-tax money for qualified medical expenses, such as cosmetic procedures that are deemed medically necessary. By utilizing HSAs or FSAs, patients can make the most of their healthcare dollars and possibly lower the amount of money they have to pay out of pocket for laser skin resurfacing. By being aware of all of their financing options and choosing the best one, patients can prioritize their skin health and aesthetic goals without worrying about money.

INSURANCE PROTECTION DURING COSMETIC OPERATIONS

Although most health insurance plans do not cover elective cosmetic procedures, including laser skin resurfacing, unless deemed medically necessary, there are some situations in which laser treatments may qualify for insurance coverage if they are prescribed to address specific medical conditions, such as severe acne scars or precancerous skin lesions. Even though laser skin resurfacing is primarily considered a cosmetic procedure aimed at enhancing skin appearance and texture, insurance coverage for such treatments is typically limited.

It is important to carefully review the terms of the insurance policy and ask about pre-authorization requirements or documentation needed to facilitate claims processing. Patients interested in exploring insurance coverage for laser skin resurfacing should speak with their healthcare provider to find out if their condition meets the requirements for medical necessity. Documentation from a dermatologist or cosmetic surgeon detailing the therapeutic benefits of laser treatment may support a case for insurance reimbursement.

Being proactive in understanding insurance policies and exploring coverage options ensures that patients can make informed decisions regarding their skincare treatments while effectively managing financial responsibilities. In situations where insurance coverage is not available, patients can investigate alternative financing options or savings strategies to cover out-of-pocket expenses associated with laser skin resurfacing.

SETTING A BUDGET FOR SKIN CARE OVER TIME

While the initial procedure addresses specific skin concerns like wrinkles, sun damage, or acne scars, ongoing skincare routines, and maintenance treatments are crucial for optimizing results and preserving skin health. Including physician-recommended skincare products in daily routines helps protect the skin from environmental damage and premature aging. Planning for long-term skin care after laser skin resurfacing is essential to maintaining and improving treatment outcomes over time.

To maintain the benefits of laser skin resurfacing, patients should budget for these skincare products as part of their long-term skincare regimen. Periodic follow-up visits with the dermatologist or cosmetic surgeon may also be required to monitor skin progress and recommend additional treatments or adjustments as needed. Post-procedure maintenance may involve the use of topical treatments, moisturizers, and sunscreens to promote healing and protect the skin from UV radiation.

In addition, patients should account for the possibility of requiring touch-up laser treatments to preserve skin clarity and smoothness over time. These treatments can help address new signs of aging or preserve results from the initial procedure. Patients can benefit from laser skin resurfacing in the long run while maintaining the health and vitality of their skin if they prioritize skincare products and follow maintenance recommendations, which will keep their skin looking young and glowing for years to come.

CHAPTER NINE

SELECTING AN ELIGIBLE SUPPLIER

INVESTIGATING CLINICS AND PROVIDERS

To ensure a safe and effective procedure, do your homework before choosing a provider or clinic for laser skin resurfacing. Start by making a list of clinics that are reputable in your area or that are recognized for having specialized knowledge in dermatological procedures.

You can obtain preliminary information by using online resources like medical directories, review platforms, and healthcare websites. Take note of the clinic's profile, services provided, and any skin treatment specializations.

Then, take a closer look at each prospective provider's background. Seek credentials, certifications, and memberships in dermatology- or cosmetic surgery-related professional organizations. These indicate that the provider has undergone training and adheres to industry standards. You should also think about the technology and equipment that each clinic has on hand. Advanced laser systems guarantee accuracy and safety during procedures, so find out what kinds of lasers are used and how effective they are in skin resurfacing treatments.

Lastly, look for recommendations and evaluations from past clients. Internet reviews can offer insightful information about the treatment process, results, and general client satisfaction with the clinic's offerings. Look for recurring compliments about the professionalism, communication, and results attained by the provider.

On the other hand, be aware of any issues or unfavorable reviews and consider bringing them up in consultations to get clarification. By doing extensive research on clinics and providers, you give yourself the power to make an informed decision that puts your safety and treatment success as your top priority.

WHAT TO QUESTION IN CONSULTATIONS

Finding the best provider for your laser skin resurfacing treatment requires consultations with potential providers. Make a list of questions you want to ask to get detailed information and evaluate each one's suitability. Start by asking about the provider's experience with laser skin resurfacing specifically. Find out how many procedures they perform annually. Find out about their success and complication rates. Knowing how experienced they are will give you confidence that they can provide safe and effective treatment.

Ask about the advantages of their selected laser system, including its efficacy in treating your skin concerns, such as wrinkles, scars, or pigmentation issues. You should also inquire about the expected downtime and recovery process following treatment, including any potential risks or side effects. By discussing the specific laser technology they use for skin resurfacing, you can better prepare yourself both physically and mentally for the procedure.

Finally, talk about the provider's approach to customized treatment plans. A customized approach based on your skin type and specific goals ensures optimal results. By asking thorough questions during consultations, you gain clarity on the treatment process and can make an informed decision regarding your provider. Make sure you understand what is included in the quoted price and inquire about any additional fees or post-treatment care recommendations.

ASSESSING EXPERIENCE AND CREDENTIALS

Several important considerations should direct your evaluation of the qualifications and experience of laser skin resurfacing providers. First, confirm the provider's medical qualifications and certifications. Look for board certification in dermatology or cosmetic surgery as this signifies specialized training and adherence to strict standards of care. Next, find out about their particular experience with laser treatments, including the number of years they have been in practice and the number of procedures they perform annually.

Look for affiliations with professional organizations related to dermatology or cosmetic procedures; these can serve as indicators of the provider's reputation within the medical community in addition to their formal credentials. Research any awards or recognitions the provider may have received; these can serve as additional evidence of their expertise and dedication to patient care.

Assessing the clinic's facilities and laser skin resurfacing technology comes next. Modern laser systems guarantee accurate treatment delivery and better patient outcomes, so find out which kinds of lasers are used and how successful they have been in producing the desired results. You should also think about the provider's approach to patient safety and comfort during procedures, including any necessary anesthetic protocols and post-procedure monitoring.

You can choose a provider who prioritizes safety, achieves excellent outcomes, and offers a positive patient experience with confidence if you thoroughly evaluate credentials and experience.

Finally, review any malpractice history or disciplinary actions against the provider. State medical boards and online databases can provide insights into any past issues that may impact your decision.

EXAMINING TESTIMONIALS AND REVIEWS FROM PATIENTS

When researching potential providers, take the time to read both positive and critical reviews to obtain a thorough understanding of their reputation and patient satisfaction levels. Patient testimonials and reviews provide priceless insights into the actual experiences of people who have undergone laser skin resurfacing with a particular provider.

Look for reviews that address the bedside manner, communication skills, and outcomes of laser skin resurfacing. Consistent themes in the feedback include satisfaction with treatment outcomes, minimal downtime, and overall improvement in skin texture and appearance. To get started, look for credible review platforms and healthcare websites where patients share their treatment experiences.

Consider how these factors align with your priorities and expectations for treatment as you read through the reviews, noting any specific concerns or areas of praise mentioned by multiple patients. For example, positive reviews may highlight the provider's attention to detail during consultations, while critical reviews may mention issues with scheduling or post-procedure care.

Furthermore, look for endorsements or comparison images posted by the provider on their website or social media accounts. These visual aids can offer more information about the revolutionary effects of laser skin resurfacing and highlight the provider's skill at producing results that look natural.

In the end, patient evaluations and testimonies are an invaluable tool for assessing the general quality of care and patient satisfaction with a laser skin resurfacing provider. By carefully considering this input, you can make a well-informed choice that is consistent with your objectives for smoother, more radiant skin.

USING YOUR GUT FEELINGS TO CHOOSE A PROVIDER

Trusting your gut when choosing a laser skin resurfacing provider is essential to a great treatment experience and the best possible outcomes. Although objective factors like credentials and patient testimonials are valuable, you should also consider how comfortable you are with the provider personally.

Start by evaluating how you are greeted, the level of professionalism in the clinic, and the provider's willingness to answer your questions and concerns during consultations or interactions with the office staff. A warm environment and open communication are signs of a provider who values patient-centered care.

The next thing to think about is how well the provider listens to your expectations and goals for laser skin resurfacing. A collaborative approach, in which the provider gives you, personalized treatment recommendations based on your particular skin concerns, shows that they are committed to helping you achieve your goals. If you feel understood and heard during these conversations, you should trust your gut.

Think about how comfortable you feel overall with the suggested course of treatment and how well the provider explains the process to you. Being open and honest about the possible dangers, advantages, and anticipated results helps you to have faith in the provider's knowledge.

Lastly, take into account any recommendations from friends or family who has had comparable treatments with the provider. These can provide extra assurance and information about the practitioner's standing in your community.

You can approach laser skin resurfacing with confidence and peace of mind by following your gut and choosing a provider who values your values and treatment goals. Your intuition is a valuable resource for helping you choose a provider who puts your safety, satisfaction, and general well-being first.

CHAPTER TEN

OPTIONS NOT INCLUDED IN LASER SKIN RESURFACING

ALTERNATIVES TO LASERS FOR SKIN RESURFACING

Non-laser options for skin resurfacing offer alternative methods to achieve smoother, more youthful skin without the use of laser technology. These alternatives include chemical peels, microdermabrasion, and dermabrasion, each targeting different skin concerns and conditions. Chemical peels involve the application of a chemical solution to the skin, which exfoliates the outer layer and promotes new skin cell growth. This treatment is effective for improving skin texture, reducing fine lines, and treating acne scars. Microdermabrasion utilizes a handheld device to gently exfoliate the skin with fine crystals or a diamond-tipped wand, buffing away dead skin cells and stimulating collagen production. It is beneficial for improving skin tone, reducing minor scars, and enhancing the absorption of skincare products. Dermabrasion, on the other hand, is a more intensive procedure that involves the mechanical removal of the outer layers of skin using a rotating brush or diamond wheel. This treatment is effective for deeper scars, wrinkles, and pigmentation issues.

Considering the pros and cons of each non-laser option, it is important to consult a skincare professional to determine which is best for your specific skin type, concerns, and desired results. Professionals can assess skin conditions, discuss treatment goals, and recommend the safest and most effective approach. Chemical peels range in intensity from superficial to deep, allowing for tailored treatments based on skin type and concerns. Microdermabrasion is non-invasive and requires minimal downtime, making it suitable for those with busy schedules. Dermabrasion, although more aggressive, provides significant results for severe skin imperfections but may require longer recovery periods.

COMPARING VARIOUS TREATMENT APPROACHES

It's important to comprehend the distinct advantages and drawbacks of each skin resurfacing treatment modality when comparing them. Chemical peels, microdermabrasion, and dermabrasion differ in technique, strength, and outcomes, meeting the needs of different skin types and concerns. Chemical peels use different acids, like glycolic, salicylic, or trichloroacetic acid, to exfoliate the skin and improve texture; they can be classified as superficial, medium, or deep peels, each providing varying degrees of exfoliation and addressing particular skin conditions like acne scars, pigmentation, and fine lines. Microdermabrasion is a mechanical exfoliation technique that uses abrasive crystals or a diamond-tipped wand to remove dead skin cells and promote collagen production.

When deciding between these modalities, people should speak with a qualified skincare professional to assess their skin condition, discuss treatment goals, and choose the best option. Professionals can provide personalized recommendations based on skin type, sensitivity, and desired outcomes, ensuring safe and effective treatment. By weighing the advantages and potential risks of each modality, people can make an informed decision to achieve the desired results. Dermabrasion is a more aggressive procedure that uses a rotating instrument to mechanically abrade the skin's surface, effectively smoothing out deeper wrinkles, scars, and pigmentation irregularities. It requires a longer recovery period compared to chemical peels and microdermabrasion but can yield dramatic results for severe skin concerns.

RECOGNIZING THEIR BENEFITS AND DRAWBACKS

Making educated decisions about skincare requires knowing the benefits and drawbacks of various skin resurfacing procedures.

Chemical peels provide customized options with different depths and formulations to target specific concerns like fine lines, acne scars, and hyperpigmentation. They encourage the production of collagen and improve skin texture, but depending on the intensity of the peel, they may cause temporary redness, peeling, or sensitivity. Microdermabrasion is a gentle exfoliation suitable for all skin types, improving product absorption and stimulating cellular renewal. It is non-invasive and requires no downtime, though it may require multiple sessions for best results. Dermabrasion, on the other hand, is more aggressive and effectively treats deeper scars and wrinkles by removing layers of skin.

A consultation with skincare professionals is necessary to determine the suitability of each treatment, taking into account factors such as skin type, medical history, and desired results. Professionals can recommend the safest and most effective option based on individual needs, ensuring optimal results with minimal risk.

People can choose a treatment that fits their lifestyle and skincare goals by weighing the pros and cons of chemical peels, microdermabrasion, and dermabrasion. They can make an informed decision by taking into consideration factors like downtime, potential side effects, and expected results.

SEEKING GUIDANCE FROM EXPERTS

For skin resurfacing procedures, seeking advice from skincare professionals is crucial to ensuring safe and effective results. Dermatologists, plastic surgeons, and licensed skincare specialists are skilled in evaluating skin conditions, suggesting appropriate treatments, and attending to individual concerns. In consultations, professionals assess skin type, texture, and any issues that may already be present, such as wrinkles, acne scars, or irregular pigmentation. They go over treatment options, including chemical peels, microdermabrasion, and dermabrasion, outlining the advantages, risks, and anticipated outcomes of each modality.

Additionally, professionals take into account medical history, allergies, and sensitivity to customize treatments to each patient's needs while minimizing potential risks.

To achieve desired results, skin care professionals may suggest a course of treatments or combination therapies. They also educate patients on pre-treatment preparation, post-care instructions, and potential side effects to promote healing and optimize results. By speaking with skincare experts, individuals can obtain important insights into the specific needs of their skin and guidance on which treatment to choose to achieve smoother, more youthful-looking skin. Professional advice guarantees a holistic approach to skincare, boosting confidence and satisfaction with treatment outcomes.

MAKING KNOWLEDGEABLE CHOICES REGARDING YOUR SKINCARE

Understanding the options for skin resurfacing and selecting the best treatment for your needs and preferences is essential to making informed skincare decisions. Chemical peels, microdermabrasion, and dermabrasion are three different ways to improve skin texture, minimize imperfections, and improve overall appearance. Chemical peels use different acids to exfoliate the skin and stimulate collagen production; depending on treatment goals and skin condition, there are options ranging from superficial to deep peels. Microdermabrasion is a gentle exfoliation method that uses abrasive crystals or a diamond-tipped wand to gently exfoliate the skin. This method is useful for improving skin tone, minimizing fine lines, and improving productivity.

To address deeper wrinkles, scars, and pigmentation issues, dermabrasion is a more intensive procedure that involves longer recovery times but yields notable improvements in skin texture and appearance. People should think about treatment goals, availability of downtime, and possible side effects when choosing skincare treatments.

CHAPTER ELEVEN

TRENDS IN SKIN RESURFACING IN THE FUTURE

DEVELOPMENTS IN LASER TECHNOLOGY

New lasers, like fractional lasers and picosecond lasers, have emerged as potent tools in dermatological practices. Fractional lasers, for example, work by targeting only a fraction of the skin's surface, leaving the surrounding tissue intact, which promotes faster healing and reduces downtime. On the other hand, picosecond lasers deliver ultra-short pulses of energy that break down pigment particles and stimulate collagen production, effectively treating pigmentation issues and improving skin texture. Recent advancements in laser technology have revolutionized skin resurfacing procedures, offering more precise and effective treatments than ever before.

Further developments in cooling systems integrated into these lasers improve patient comfort during procedures, making skin resurfacing more tolerable and accessible to a wider range of patients. Dermatologists can now more accurately tailor treatments to individual skin types and concerns, minimizing the risk of adverse effects and maximizing treatment efficacy. Such advancements in technology have also led to the development of laser systems with improved safety profiles and customizable treatment parameters.

The ongoing advancement of laser technology in skin resurfacing has raised the bar for dermatological care considerably. These innovations have been shown to improve treatment outcomes as well as patient satisfaction by minimizing discomfort and downtime.

Going forward, dermatologists can anticipate further improvements in laser systems, which will open the door to even more accessible and effective skin rejuvenation treatments.

NEW METHODOLOGIES AND INNOVATIONS

New advances in laser skin resurfacing concentrate on improving treatment accuracy, safety, and effectiveness. One noteworthy development is the merging of lasers with other modalities, like ultrasound and radiofrequency, to produce synergistic effects that target multiple skin layers for all-encompassing skin rejuvenation. This strategy enables dermatologists to treat a greater variety of skin issues, such as wrinkles and fine lines, acne scars, and hyperpigmentation, in a single session.

Furthermore, advancements in pulse control technology allow dermatologists to more precisely adjust laser parameters, ensuring optimal treatment outcomes while minimizing the risk of side effects. Fractional ablative laser resurfacing is another promising technique, delivering microscopic columns of laser energy to the skin, stimulating collagen production, and promoting faster healing compared to traditional ablative lasers.

Advances in laser resurfacing have also been extended to handheld devices for use at home; these, however, usually offer tamer treatments more appropriate for maintenance than intense rejuvenation. Frequently, these devices use light-based technologies to target particular skin concerns, giving users easy choices for maintaining their skin in between professional treatments.

New methods and advancements in laser skin resurfacing are enhancing treatment options and enhancing patient outcomes for skin rejuvenation. Dermatologists can set new benchmarks for minimally invasive cosmetic procedures by fusing cutting-edge technologies and optimizing treatment protocols to produce more consistent results with fewer side effects.

PROSPECTIVE ADVANTAGES OF NOVEL ADVANCEMENTS

The most recent advancements in laser skin resurfacing have the potential to benefit patients and dermatologists alike. Enhanced accuracy and effectiveness allow treatments to target particular skin concerns more effectively, such as diminishing wrinkles, enhancing skin texture, or fading pigmentation irregularities. These developments also translate into shorter recovery times and less discomfort following the procedure, enabling patients to resume their daily activities sooner.

Newer laser technologies also frequently have improved safety features and programmable settings, which reduce the possibility of negative reactions and guarantee a customized approach to each patient's particular skin type and condition. This degree of personalization not only results in better treatment outcomes but also increases patient satisfaction with more consistent and natural-looking results.

The benefits of these advancements from the standpoint of a dermatologist are greater treatment versatility and efficiency. With better instruments at their disposal, practitioners can broaden the scope of services they offer and treat a more diverse patient base with a range of skin concerns. This can result in higher patient retention rates and a stronger reputation for providing outstanding cosmetic outcomes.

The future of skin rejuvenation appears bright, with further advancements likely to further refine and expand the capabilities of laser-based treatments. The potential benefits of new developments in laser skin resurfacing are numerous, promising improved treatment precision, enhanced safety, and greater patient satisfaction.

CONSUMER PREFERENCES AND INDUSTRY TRENDS

This shift toward non-surgical solutions has driven innovation in laser technologies, leading to the development of more sophisticated devices that cater to these preferences. Current industry trends in laser skin resurfacing reflect a growing demand for non-invasive procedures that deliver natural-looking results with minimal downtime.

Patients are increasingly seeking treatments that offer both immediate improvements and long-term benefits, such as collagen stimulation and skin texture refinement.

Additionally, a trend toward combination therapies—combining laser resurfacing with other modalities such as injectables or topical skincare products—is evident. These synergistic approaches offer complete skin rejuvenation by addressing various aging and skin damage aspects in a single treatment session, emphasizing the value of customized treatment plans that take into account each patient's particular concerns and aesthetic goals.

When it comes to laser skin resurfacing treatments, consumer preferences also prioritize safety, efficacy, and affordability. New developments in laser technology that provide better results with fewer side effects are appealing to discerning patients who value safety and results equally. Package deals and financing options also make these treatments more accessible to a wider range of people, which is driving market growth.

As these trends continue to develop, dermatologists and aesthetic practitioners can anticipate ongoing innovation in laser technologies and treatment protocols to better serve their patients. In summary, industry trends in laser skin resurfacing highlight a shift towards holistic treatment approaches and advanced technologies that meet consumer demands for effective, safe, and convenient solutions.

MAINTAINING KNOWLEDGE AND EDUCATION FOR UPCOMING THERAPIES

For dermatologists, continuing education and training ensures proficiency in using new laser technologies and understanding their applications for various skin types and conditions. Continuing education courses and workshops offer opportunities to learn about emerging techniques, hone treatment skills, and stay up to date on best practices in dermatological care.

For patients, on the other hand, staying informed and educated about the latest developments in laser skin resurfacing is imperative.

Patient education materials and online resources have advanced, enabling consumers to make informed decisions about their skincare journey, from initial consultations to post-procedural care. Patients can stay informed by researching treatment options, comprehending the benefits and potential risks of laser skin resurfacing, and consulting with qualified practitioners who can provide personalized recommendations based on individual needs.

Dermatologists can also learn from each other, share experiences, and stay up to date on industry developments by continuing to collaborate with peers in the field. Professional associations and conferences offer forums for dermatologists to discuss the latest research findings, debate treatment approaches, and discuss potential directions for laser technology and cosmetic dermatology.

By embracing lifelong learning and being proactive in adopting new technologies, dermatologists can continue to provide safe, effective, and state-of-the-art treatments that meet the changing needs of their patients. Remaining informed and educated about advancements in laser skin resurfacing is essential for fostering innovation, improving patient outcomes, and advancing the field of cosmetic dermatology.

www.ingramcontent.com/pod-product-compliance
Lightning Source LLC
Chambersburg PA
CBHW061247250726

48653CB00002B/544